Another Bethesda Miracle

Another Bethesda Miracle

How Community, Persistence and Faith
Triumphed Over a Stroke

Bernie Oldenkamp

[signature]

DeForest Press URBAN CHURCH
Elk River, Minnesota LEADERSHIP CENTER
3000 Leonard NE - 2nd Level/GRTS
Grand Rapids, MI 49525

Copyright © 2005 by Bernard R. Oldenkamp. All rights reserved.
Published 2005.

No part of this book may be reproduced or transmitted in any form or by any means, electronic or mechanical, including photocopying, recording or by any information storage and retrieval system, without written permission from the author.

Permission gratefully acknowledged for the photos and article from the Mille Lacs County Times, ECM Publishers, Inc.

Scripture quotations are taken from the Holy Bible, New Living Translation, copyright © 1996. Used by permission of Tyndale House Publishers, Inc., Wheaton, Illinois 60189. All rights reserved.

Published by:
DeForest Press
P.O. Box 154
Elk River, MN 55330 USA
www.DeForestPress.com
Toll-free: 877-441-9733
Richard DeForest Erickson, Publisher
Shane Groth, President

Cover design by Anthony Alex LeTourneau

Library of Congress Cataloging-in-Publication Data

Oldenkamp, Bernie, 1943-
 Another Bethesda miracle : how community, persistence and faith triumphed over a stroke / By Bernie Oldenkamp.
   p. cm.
 ISBN 1-930374-21-6
 1. Cerebrovascular disease--Popular works. I. Title.
 RC388.5.O53 2005
 362.196'810092--dc22
            2005030088

To

my daughter, Marceea,
now a super mom with the Milton Hershey
Foundation, overseeing twelve teenage girls at a
group home in Pennsylvania.

my son, Jeffery,
a machinist in Fridley, Minnesota.

my son, David,
my former little bookworm boy,
and new college professor at Indiana University
in Bloomington, Indiana.

my daughter, Laura,
a park ranger in the Minnesota state park system.

my wife, Imogene (Irons) Oldenkamp,
a woman of boundless energy, courage and
compassion—the take-charge type.

Contents

Acknowledgments 8
1 Rise and Crash 11
2 Angels Day and Night 18
3 The Milaca Factor 21
4 The Upgrade 30
5 Moving Day 34
6 The Sore Nurse 37
7 The Spanish Factor 41
8 Occupational, Physical & Speech Therapy 43
9 A Christmas Visit 62
10 A Miracle 64
11 The "61" Factor 68
12 Living with a Stroke 71
13 Mud and Mail 73
14 A Tractor Ride 76
15 Conrad Winslow 78
16 Saudades 80
17 A Visitor's View 81
18 To My Students 85
19 The Faith Factor 90

Acknowledgments

My thanks to Lola Murphy and Imogene Oldenkamp for their keyboard skills, to Dawn Slade for her encouragement and support, and to Tony LeTourneau for his illustration and cover design.

Also, a huge expression of thanks goes to the Tim and Donelle Welch family for the hands that have helped along the way, not the least of which was the fishing outing at the "cabin."

Afterward Jesus returned to Jerusalem for one of the Jewish holy days. Inside the city, near the Sheep Gate, was the pool of Bethesda, with five covered porches. Crowds of sick people—blind, lame, or paralyzed—lay on the porches. One of the men lying there had been sick for thirty-eight years. When Jesus saw him and knew how long he had been ill, he asked him, "Would you like to get well?"

"I can't, sir," the sick man said, "for I have no one to help me into the pool when the water is stirred up."

Jesus told him, "Stand up, pick up your sleeping mat, and walk!" (John 5:1-7a, 8a, NLT).

Chapter One

Rise and Crash

It's a sixty-mile trek one way from our little house in the big woods east of Hinckley, Minnesota, to the elementary school parking lot in front of the Milaca Elementary School in Milaca, Minnesota. For five years, without missing one day, I had made the daily journey without incident. I was always on time as a bus driver for the 6:50 A.M. route beginning in Bock, Minnesota, and ending at the elementary school in Milaca for the 8:05 A.M. start of my day as a teacher.

My daily teaching schedule started at 8:30 A.M. in the Spanish classroom. Every student from first

ANOTHER BETHESDA MIRACLE

grade through sixth grade would come to my room for a half-hour Spanish class twice a week.

On the morning of October 16, 2001, my little alarm clock didn't look the same at 4 A.M. when I woke up. I couldn't see the hands on the face; at least, I couldn't tell where they were pointing. I had a slight headache; I just didn't feel quite right. My wife, Imogene, urged me to get going because breakfast was ready. But I wasn't.

When I did appear at the kitchen table at 4:15 A.M., I had my T-shirt on backwards and inside out. Imogene suggested I go back and start over. I could walk and talk fine, so I had no warning anything was seriously wrong with me. I had taken my shower, found two aspirin, and took my prescribed blood pressure pills. I waited a few minutes for the headache to pass, but the clock kept ticking. I needed to be on the road at 5:30 A.M. sharp. By 6:00 A.M. I'm normally at Hinckley, twenty miles away, and by 6:40 A.M. I'm rolling out the "Flower Bus" (number 61) for the pre-trip inspection at Sue's Bus Company in Bock.

My wife had turned the Buick Park Avenue around for me and had pointed it down the driveway. I headed out. I thought the cool, fresh October air would wake me up. The first twenty miles on my daily trip are on State Highway 48, heading west toward Hinckley. It turns out, I was on the road to disaster, and later, a miracle.

Only later, after my accident, I was informed that I had been driving on the wrong side of the highway with drivers coming toward me, heading for the ditch to the left of me. I had gone past three churches and five bridges, but I don't remember going by anything. Apparently someone had alerted the state patrol because they were waiting for me in Hinckley, but I never arrived.

Just prior to the accident, I do remember a school bus heading toward me. I can still see the clip lights, three of them, above the windshield and one on each side. The bus had its headlights on. All of a sudden the bus was right in front of me. The crash was loud. There was a loud burst in my car, the airbag exploding like a shotgun blast.

I remember seeing the driver of the bus take a bounce. Fortunately, there were no children on the bus. And no one was riding with me. The state patrol arrived quickly with their lights flashing. I do remember the fire truck, but not a fire. I started yelling. I also remember comforting voices. I knew one voice was that of Skip, a man from my church. (He has been with the fire department for many years). The other familiar voice was a Hinckley High School teacher.

I was trapped inside my car. I still don't know which fireman actually worked the Jaws of Life extractor-cutting machine. They proceeded to cut the doorpost off at the roof level (by my left ear) and tried to get the door open. They ended up cutting off the car door. All this time I was yelling. I knew I would be late for school.

I told the state patrol officer to call my wife and the Milaca district office. The elementary school office needed to know what had happened. I rattled off the phone numbers. They also needed to call the bus garage in Bock. Not knowing how seriously I was injured, I thought I would be late for work or perhaps need a substitute. (The sub folder was on my desk).

The emergency crew somehow got a wide, smooth board under me from the right side and got me out of the car. My chest and upper body really hurt. I still don't know how I found so much air for all of this talking and yelling! I did not know until months later that many of my ribs were broken and my lungs had collapsed and had been punctured. I also was unaware at the time that I was bleeding internally. The state patrol report would later reveal that the pavement was dry at the time of the accident. There were no skid marks. Apparently I did not even apply the brakes before I hit the bus head-on.

The Pine County ambulance from Hinckley headed for Mora, Minnesota, at my request. I don't remember much about that twenty miles, but I

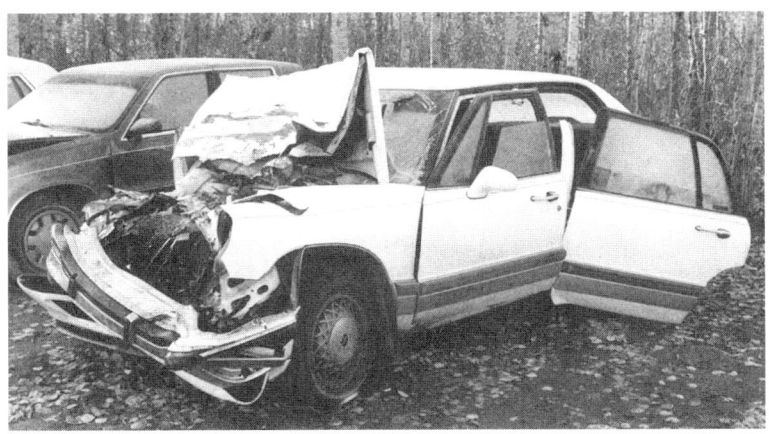

Bernie's car after the accident

Rise and Crash

did ask Skip, the attendant, if we had gone past Quamba, Minnesota, yet. I knew every crossroad and curve on State Highway 23.

That morning, my wife, Imogene, had been driving her regular school bus route. Her friends, Shar, Randy and Jack, were at the Fleming Logging Road waiting for her as she arrived with the school bus. They stopped her and asked Imogene to get out of the bus. Mr. Almos confirmed there had been an accident.

Randy took my wife to Mora to meet the ambulance. Randy is a road construction worker who was staying with us while he was working nearby. He got permission from his boss to go find Imogene on the bus route and later came upon the accident.

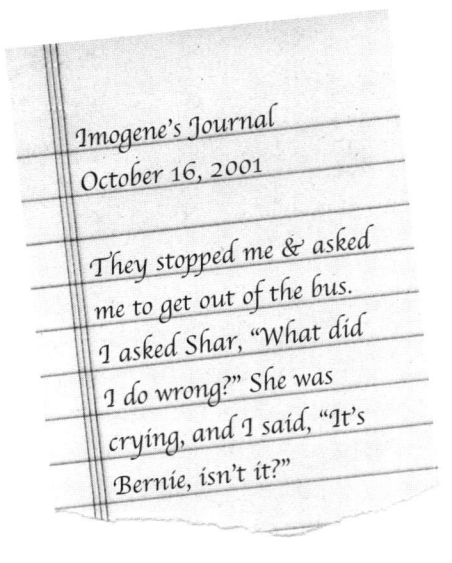

> *Imogene's Journal*
> *October 16, 2001*
>
> *They stopped me & asked me to get out of the bus.*
> *I asked Shar, "What did I do wrong?" She was crying, and I said, "It's Bernie, isn't it?"*

In Mora, a Life Link chopper was waiting on the pad and, with a quick transfer, I was bound for North Memorial Trauma Center in Minneapolis. My next thirty days are blank. I was unconscious for about a month. My wife, Imogene, kept a journal of those days while I was "out of it." Apparently a flurry of phone calls and bleak reports triggered

ANOTHER BETHESDA MIRACLE

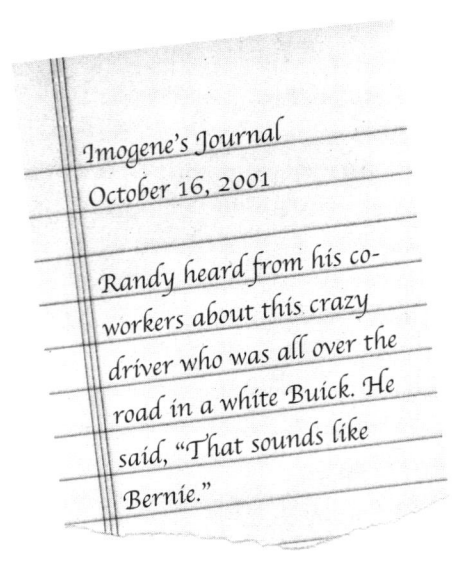

> *Imogene's Journal*
> *October 16, 2001*
>
> *Randy heard from his co-workers about this crazy driver who was all over the road in a white Buick. He said, "That sounds like Bernie."*

friends and family to visit me at intensive care at North Memorial.

My brothers Bill and J.B. drove from Michigan to see me. One of them told the other that he wouldn't lay down a "plug nickel" to ever see me up and around again. They listened to the doctor in charge, gave Imogene a hug and went out the door, shaking their heads.

The doctor did his best to prepare Imogene for the tough reality of my situation. I had internal bleeding, a punctured lung, a bruised heart, a broken right leg above the ankle, and my left hand had apparently hit the windshield pretty hard. I was given two pints of blood because of my internal bleeding. I did eventually see the hospital bill for severing the last remaining tendon on my left pointer finger. What was a finger is now a stub. It would be a month later before I would even know it was missing. Yellow jaundice, pneumonia and a stomach ulcer were later added to my list of woes. My doctor said perhaps the amount of medicine I was given may have triggered some of my problems.

Rise and Crash

The first time I remember seeing my left hand, it was full of ugly black stitches and red, orange, yellow, blue, purple, and green skin. I was unable to move my hand until Imogene spent a few days and nights working it over, doing the "milk-the-cow" routine. Slowly the natural color came back to my hand. A nurse had asked Imogene if she had ever milked a cow before. A dumb question. At a farm in Tillamook, Oregon, she milked 400 Holsteins before 7:00 A.M. in the milking parlor with a Mexican helper. She sat by my bed day and night squeezing and rubbing from my fingertips through my palm and towards my elbow.

Even a month into my slow recovery, my problems persisted and new ones developed. For example, my nervous system could not handle noise. I had watched just twenty minutes of a professional football game one Sunday afternoon while every TV on the hospital floor was on full blast. This really got to me, so I rarely watched any television at all. I slowly adjusted to my new situation.

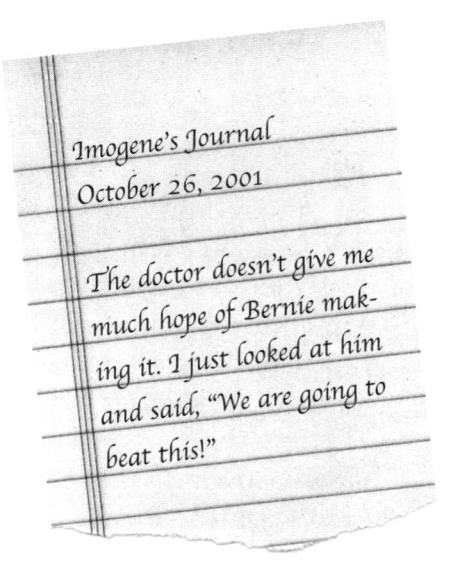

> *Imogene's Journal*
> *October 26, 2001*
>
> The doctor doesn't give me much hope of Bernie making it. I just looked at him and said, "We are going to beat this!"

Chapter Two

Angels Day and Night

My month-long intensive care experience at North Memorial was mostly a blur. Imogene was there at my side almost every day, but I don't remember it. Although I had many, many visitors, I only clearly recall one visitor while I was in intensive care. A tall, slender man appeared one afternoon at my door. He had on a dress shirt and tie. He walked slowly towards me, took my right hand and said, "Let's pray." It was a beautiful experience. My visitor was Dr. Steven Keillor, historian and author from Askov, Minnesota. I was a first- and second-grade teacher to his two sons, Will and Jeremy.

Other visitors included a dear pastor and his wife from Green Isle, Minnesota. They would stand by the bedside and sing softly and pray. They would hold my hand and I felt their healing presence. Imogene said they came to visit about every week. Dear pastor friends from St. James, Minnesota, would also appear weekly to sing and pray.

Imogene tried to keep a daily log of phone calls and visitors, but this was difficult because there were so many. She finally resorted to a piece of tag board, plastered on the closet door, where my visitors could sign their names, kind of like a guest book.

The angels kept coming even after my move to Bethesda. Well after visiting hours one night two men tapped quietly on my door and came in. I don't know how they got past security at that hour. One of the visitors was my dear friend John, fresh from working all day on the Soo Railroad line in Superior, Wisconsin. Fresh from the bush country of Markville, Minnesota, the other fella was Larry, paralyzed from the waist down, cruising along in a wheelchair. How refreshing! They prayed long and hard.

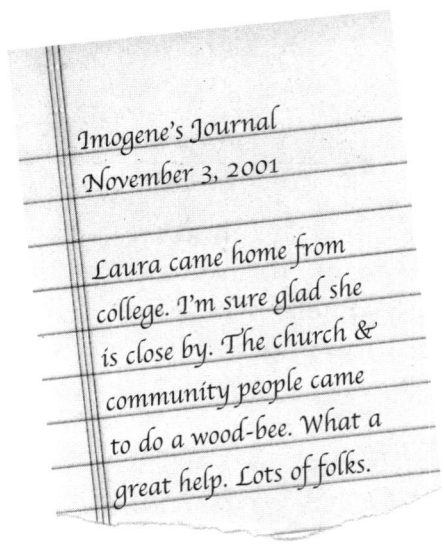

> *Imogene's Journal*
> *November 3, 2001*
>
> *Laura came home from college. I'm sure glad she is close by. The church & community people came to do a wood-bee. What a great help. Lots of folks.*

ANOTHER BETHESDA MIRACLE

One very dreary December afternoon I was feeling really low. Couldn't anyone come see me? I cried inwardly. My door began to move, and in came a former student of mine. It was Magen, now a college student in Eau Clarie. I went to pieces and slobbered all over her nice leather jacket.

With every visit more healing came. I felt myself getting stronger in body, mind and spirit. To me, these people who came to my bedside, known and unknown, were angels. They were sweet-spirited people on a mission with a quiet and determined message of love and hope. God bless them all!

> *Visitor's note*
>
> *Hey, Bernie,*
> *Me and John come down to tell ya we care and we love ya and we are praying for ya,*
>
> *Love, Larry Holman*

Chapter Three

The Milaca Factor

I will be forever grateful for the visits to the hospital from Ann Kern, the principal and my boss at Milaca Elementary School. I also deeply appreciated the delivery of a huge poster signed by over 600 students and school staff. The hospital staff had never seen such a large poster with so many names.

A mountain of mail arrived at the hospital during October, November, and December as teachers and entire classes kept the postal service in business with messages of hope and cheer. I loved every

ANOTHER BETHESDA MIRACLE

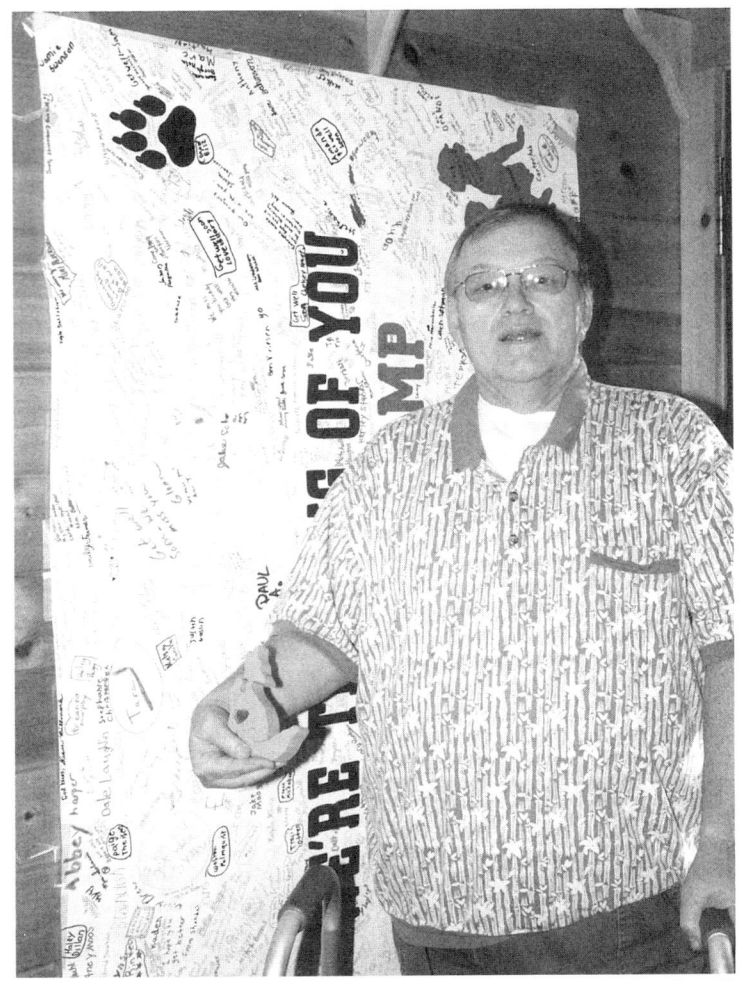

Bernie and the poster signed by over 600 students and school staff

card and letter. Folks from the Milaca community also sent notes and letters of encouragement.

The Milaca school staff aided in my recovery effort. Their "Sunshine Committee" collected a nice sum of money and put it in Imogene's hand one day at the hospital. We were truly blessed.

The Milaca Factor

The Milaca community also was very generous with their support. The parent-teacher group from the community planned a fundraiser dinner that was held after I was released from the hospital. The Sunday afternoon taco dinner brought nearly 1,000 people to the high school cafeteria for the dinner and raffle. What a crew! Thanks to the sixth graders for serving! I'm still overwhelmed as I write this.

After getting home again, a small group of teachers with big hearts came to my home one evening with a kettle of soup and fresh bread. What a treat!

Dawn Slade from the Milaca County Times came to our house and wrote a feature story on my accident and recovery. I truly appreciated her

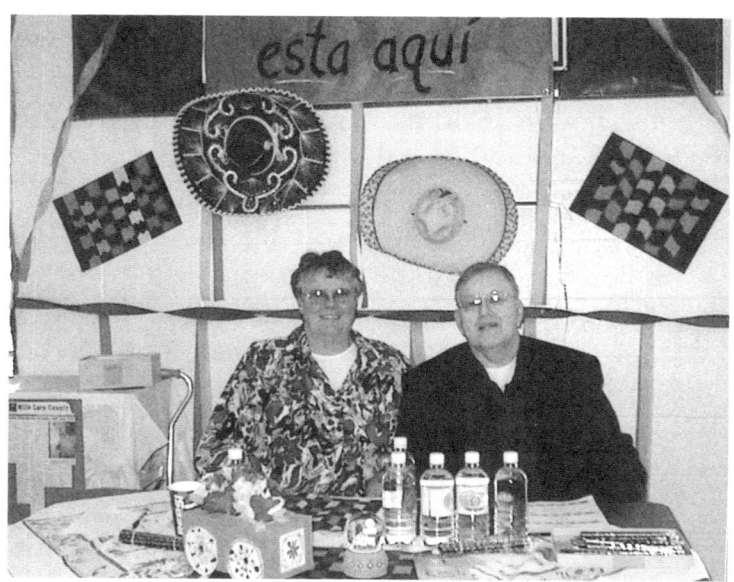

Imogene and Bernie at taco dinner fundraiser

kindness and writings. Here's the article in its entirety.

There were a few minor signals that something was wrong, but Bernie Oldenkamp, a Spanish teacher at Milaca Elementary, didn't recognize them in time.

On October 16, 2001, Oldenkamp, who lives east of Hinckley, was on the way to his bus route in Bock (he drives school bus before teaching Spanish in Milaca). During that morning drive, Oldenkamp had a stroke. His car swerved back and forth and eventually hit a school bus.

The Hinckley Fire Department used the jaws of life to remove Oldenkamp. While the crews were working, Oldenkamp recalls how he informed emergency personnel of all the people they needed to call and all their telephone numbers.

The Pine County Ambulance brought him to Mora Hospital. The last thing Oldenkamp remembers during that ambulance ride, was asking the driver, Skip, if they had gone by Quamba yet.

From the Mora Hospital he was immediately transferred by helicopter to North Memorial Hospital in Robbinsdale. Oldenkamp had suffered a broken right leg, a broken sternum, broken ribs on both sides, a bruised heart, and a punctured lung, which eventually collapsed.

The Milaca Factor

Oldenkamp's left hand had gone through the windshield and his right index finger was amputated at the hospital.

Doctors later informed Oldenkamp that when he had arrived at the hospital, he was bleeding internally and was just minutes away from death. He was in intensive care for a month.

While at North Memorial, Oldenkamp ended up having another surgery (he unknowingly pulled tubes out), he recovered from a bleeding ulcer and suffered through pneumonia.

The only thing Oldenkamp remembers about that month was Steve Keillor coming into his room, grabbing his hand and telling Oldenkamp, "Let's pray."

A doctor at North Memorial told Oldenkamp that he would be spending the rest of his life in a nursing home. Oldenkamp's wife, Imogene (Emma) wouldn't stand for that. "Oh no, we're going to beat this thing," she told them.

A month after the accident, Oldenkamp was transferred to Bethesda Lutheran Hospital and Rehabilitation Center in St. Paul.

He spent the rest of November, all of December and a few days in January working on going home.

Oldenkamp said his students might be happy to learn that he had to take a lot of tests while going through therapy. He went through physical therapy, occupational therapy and speech therapy. Part of that therapy included tests in reading comprehension, math and organization skills.

Because he couldn't put weight on his left leg, the doctors hoisted Oldenkamp up in what he refers to as a "bungie machine," so he could practice walking in place.

Oldenkamp didn't think he'd ever walk again, but he's learned to use both a walker and a cane. Doctors were surprised at his recovery and told Oldenkamp that he either met or exceeded all of their expectations. So, on Jan. 5, Oldenkamp finally went home.

He's still going to therapy weekly but says, "I want to be back in the classroom."

And by the number of cards, posters and messages Oldenkamp has received, he is greatly missed by the students and staff who want him back as well. Stacks of cards from kids with well wishes, some in Spanish, bring a smile to Oldenkamp's face.

Donelle Welch, a teacher at Milaca Elementary, said, "Señor Oldenkamp teaches Spanish across the hall from my kindergarten classroom. I have greatly enjoyed being 'neighbors' with him. He is very well liked by the the students, parents and staff here in Milaca. Señor Oldenkamp

The Milaca Factor

is a motivating teacher. He doesn't teach in a traditional way. He speaks in Spanish to the class and they learn by doing.

"One day he spoke in Spanish telling one child in each of his classes to pour a cup of water over his head. Each child knew exactly what he was instructing them to do, so they did it!

"I hear a lot of Spanish spoken, a lot of laughter and a lot of active learning going on in his classroom. Sometimes he even falls out of his chair in excitement when the children are able to count to 100 in Spanish.

"It hasn't been the same for the children here at Milaca Elementary School. He is missed greatly. We are all hoping and praying for his fast and complete recovery. He is a friendly guy, with a big heart."

The "Sunshine Committee," a group of staff members at the school, quickly came to the aid of Oldenkamp. Just two days after his accident, the staff gave him $1,250. The money was used to help replace the car that was totalled in the accident.

Before he could leave the hospital, one of his "tests" was to see if he could get in and out of the new car. Oldenkamp accomplished that task and proudly says, "No one needs to help me with my peg leg."

The Milaca Elementary staff and the Parent and Teacher Organization are planning a community fundraiser/benefit (a taco supper) to help with the many medical expenses Oldenkamp has.

Oldenkamp has come a long way since October 16. He's lost 50 pounds since the accident, but jokingly warns, "Don't try the crash diet."

He says he loves getting calls and visitors and is very appreciative of his "Milaca" family.

Strokes can cause bouts of depression and during one of his "pity parties," as Oldenkamp puts it, a letter arrived from a parent of one of his students. In part of her letter, Beth Watson says, "I know of no other person that has made such an impact on our son. He simply adores you." Watson told the *Times* that her son thinks of Mr. Oldenkamp every night in his prayers.

Oldenkamp is eager to return to the classroom and is trying to figure out how he can throw his annual piñata party for all 28 classes.

Oldenkamp has taught Spanish to over 650 students at Milaca Elementary for five years.

Prior to teaching at Milaca, Oldenkamp learned to speak Portuguese on the streets of Brazil, he worked in the Peace Corps for three years and then spent five years with a mission.

He has taught school in Alaska and Oregon, at Harvest Christian School in Sandstone, and at Nah-Ya-Shing in Onamia.

Oldenkamp wants the students to know he's fine, but that he may not be quite the same person when he returns to the classroom. He says he's going to work at having more patience.

"When life throws you a curve, you can get bitter or get better. I choose to get better," Oldenkamp says. "And I want to thank everyone who has helped me get better."

And finally, one more blessing from the teachers. When my disability paperwork was all in place, my income barely covered the mortgage. My Blue Cross health insurance through the school was good, but now I had to pay my own health insurance because I was no longer teaching. I explained this predicament to one of the teachers. Within one week I received an envelope with $340; my monthly bill in the district office was $338. Another miracle!

The goodness of God was certainly shown to me and my family through the kindness of the Milaca community. Words cannot thank them enough and I will never forget their acts of love and healing.

Chapter Four

The Upgrade

Imogene was determined to get another car because my dear Buick Park Avenue was a total loss. She said that she had prayed about getting another Buick. She loved that car. The Chevy dealer in Hinckley informed her when she started looking around for a car that he had a '92 "Caddy" that might fill the bill.

Unbeknown to us, our son, David, at Syracuse University in New York, had started an email fundraiser (a plea via email) to his college buddies from Arkansas for the "Car Fund." Within a few days checks began arriving at home from

The Upgrade

unknown addresses. Family, friends, and church folks continued sending money. Within two weeks Imogene had enough money in hand to close the deal on the nice, used '92 "Caddy." I kept telling those who would listen that she had prayed for a Buick, but the good Lord had an upgrade in mind.

Imogene waited a few days before giving me the big news from Milaca about the chunk of money from the Sunshine Committee. She was without wheels and was depending on others to get her back and forth to the hospital. Bless Bill Loomis for all of the rides he provided for her.

One afternoon Imogene came to Bethesda, pulled the curtain, and said, "Look, Dad, there it is—the gray one on top of that ramp. Our '92 'Caddy.' The Lord upgraded us. We had enough money. Can you imagine us dirt-poor farmers/school teacher riding around in that?" The money just kept coming. God is good all the time.

While I was in my hospital bed, I often wondered what everyone was thinking about me. Would they still have nursing home on the agenda? Some would come and look at me and wonder out loud if I would ever rise up again. The Lord and I had a good chat. I don't make deals with God. He now had me where he wanted me, down, but not out. I could still move my right side, so I'd have to work on those muscles and deal with the left side whenever possible.

Each day at North Memorial a brain nurse (a nurse psychologist—or whoever came with her) would approach my bed ever so quietly and ask me the same questions: "Mr. Oldenkamp, where are you now? What day is it?" I supposed they wanted to figure out how much of a brain I had left.

One day the medication nurse came to my room after breakfast and cheerfully announced that she had a new pill for me to take. I asked what it was. She said, "It's Ritalin; it will help your brain make better connections." I replied, "Well, if it will get me off the ceiling at night it would be worth a try."

That very day a group of teachers came from Milaca. I asked them to gather around my bed because I had a very important announcement. I said, "You know how they have those special meetings with the nurse and parents at school when a child goes on Ritalin? Well, they just put the teacher on Ritalin." It did help. I could tell the difference.

I couldn't wait until November 11. The day finally arrived. When the nurse asked me, on November 11, 2001, what day it was, I replied, " It's the eleventh hour of the eleventh day of the eleventh month. Now why don't you take an eleven-minute break?" In about fifteen minutes the nurse came back with another pill. Instead of one Ritalin per day, I would be taking two. My mouth

> *Imogene's Journal*
>
> Some of the teachers or staff from Milaca came to the hospital. It's so nice to have them come—the days get really long down here.

The Upgrade

was going to get me in more trouble if I didn't tone things down a bit. The nurse didn't appreciate my sense of humor.

I remembered something else about November 11. Mr. Bostic, our former superintendent, patrolled the hallways at the Milaca elementary school every November 11 in full military uniform, including his medals of honor for service to our country. He picked up every scrap of paper he saw on the floor. When the announcements started at 8:20 A.M. with the pledge of allegiance, everyone was to be in their rooms with their hand on their heart.

About every day they would ask the name of the president of the United States. I would often feel a campaign speech coming on, so they backed off on that one.

They also gave me problems to figure out, like this one: "Jay is taller than Sue. Mary is shorter than Jay. Alice is taller than Mary. So, Mr. Oldenkamp, put these in order from tallest to shortest." I repeated back the names in what I thought was the correct order. The man who asked the question leaned his head on the bed rail, shook his head and said, "I've been here eight years and no one has ever got this right." I had nailed it, and those were not even my favorite problems in math. So I guess I had some brain left.

How is your brain today? The rehab doctor's favorite teaser for me was to count backwards by sevens, starting at 100. For example, 100, 93, 86, 79, 72, 65, 58, 51, 44, 37, 30, 23, 16, 9, 2. If you're thinking about having a stroke, you can start practicing this exercise now.

Chapter Five

Moving Day

Someone told me that I was going to be moved on November 16, but that I was not going home. The big debate seemed to be whether or not I could be rehabilitated or if I belonged in a nursing home. When nursing home was mentioned, I said to myself, "Just a minute here; I don't think so." They decided to send me to Bethesda Lutheran Hospital in Saint Paul for rehabilitation.

On the eve of the transfer, the main doctor at intensive care came up with the idea to put a "bird's nest" in somewhere around my belly button in some main veins coming from my legs. This nest device is supposed to catch blood clots before they travel to my lungs or heart. Sounded like a plan. I'd been playing with bird nests ever since childhood, even collecting them from the swamps and bushy areas in the autumn after the leaves had fallen. A mechanical lift was used to lift me out of bed and onto a gurney, which raced me down a hall and elevator into a surgery room. I remember the ceiling lights were really moving overhead. My ribs still hurt with the slightest movement. In surgery I was given my "bird's nest."

This wasn't my first surgery, of course. I learned that I had made an earlier trip to surgery because I had pulled drainage tubes out of my sides, tubes that were draining blood into a bucket or two because of internal bleeding. That, apparently, was a "no-no" and the staff had to tie my hand down so I wouldn't pull that trick again. Later, they would have to tie me down again when I got to the respiratory floor at Bethesda.

I still wondered how they were going to move me. I couldn't stand or even take a step. My right leg was broken, my left leg and side was paralyzed, my sternum and many ribs were broken. There were horizontal black and blue stripes on the front of my shoulders, probably from the seatbelt. And my heart was bruised.

My questions were answered on moving day. The transfer ambulance had to have been from the Korean War. It had a three-fourths-ton chaise with no springs, plus a diesel engine, no less. And I

ANOTHER BETHESDA MIRACLE

remember billows of fumes coming up through the floorboards or lack thereof.

I immediately begged for oxygen. I asked the attendant why they would want to fumigate me now, especially after trying and succeeding to keep me alive for a month. No response; just a memorable, bumpy ride. I asked him how many miles and how long it would take from North Memorial to Bethesda in St. Paul, next to the Minnesota State Capitol. The answer, "About thirty minutes."

I also asked, "Does this Bethesda place have a pool?" I had heard of Bethesda before and recognized the name as a place in the Bible where a crippled man received healing by Jesus. Later, I would look up this account in the book of John, chapter five, when Jesus asked the paralyzed man, "Do you want to get healed?" Wow, I could use some healing.

As I bounced along on the trip across town to St. Paul, I kept worrying if my attendant would take me to the third floor balcony above the pool, open the gate and push me over the edge. He told me he had no knowledge of an actual pool at Bethesda.

I was met by a welcoming committee at Bethesda. My wife was in my new room along with very dear friends from Hinckley who were pastors at a church in St. James, Minnesota. They held my hands, sang softly and prayed long and intensely for my recovery. It was like the pool waters began to stir. Jesus, I wanted healing. Would I ever be able to stand again and take a few steps? Or would the bed be my resting place before the grave?

Chapter Six

The Sore Nurse

After just a few days at Bethesda, the bath nurses' aides were doing their thing when one of them remarked that I had a sore on my backside in the "southern hemisphere." You would think it was a major discovery. Why had I been transferred to this hospital with a sore, and no one knew about it? There seemed to be a head nurse for everything—one for blood pressure, one for the brain, one for the broken bones, and one for stomach, heart, lungs, food, and bowel movements. There was strict measuring of all fluids, in and out.

ANOTHER BETHESDA MIRACLE

By late morning, the head sore nurse was rapping on my door, which I always asked to be closed because I couldn't handle the hall noise and the vacuum sweepers. It wasn't just the head sore nurse, though. In a neat little line, each carrying a shiny little ruler, nurses kept coming into my room. She introduced herself and informed me that she had brought a group of student nurses in for the exam as part of their training. Of course, I was elated. My wife had just arrived also from her morning bus run ninety miles north.

The head sore nurse asked for some student nurses with big muscles; they were from West Africa and spoke Swahili. They did their little chant and, before I knew it, I was flipped over for all to see the area of concern.

Now, my wife is not one to be crowded out. Imogene joined them in checking me out. Years ago, she had bound my wounds and sewed up my shirts and umpiring uniforms in Alaska and Oregon where I umpired little league baseball and girls fast-pitch softball. She had not only stitched up any rips in the uniform or protective gear, but also was instrumental in lending that moral support from behind the screen when I'd make a close call. She usually hung onto the extra game ball and always had one ready in case the ball bag was empty.

When the nursing department thought they had seen enough from every angle possible, front and back, they started for the door. Then I heard this very familiar voice saying rather loudly, "Well, look! There is a hole in the ball bag!"

The Sore Nurse

After a good laugh, I said, "Now, honey, they probably call it by a more technical, scientific term around here."

The agenda at Bethesda called for a period of time in the respiratory unit, taking oxygen day and night to get me on room air. They were always checking the oxygen level in my blood.

My nights on the respiratory floor were miserable. Every night the respiratory crew strapped a mask on me from which I was to get oxygen. At first it was hard, cracked, and didn't fit over my nose correctly. I was not allowed to breathe from my mouth. If I did, an alarm would go off out in the hall, in the nurse's area. If the oxygen level in my blood got below ninety-six, another alarm would go off. I had to lay just right and not move. Certain respiratory people, male and female, would really "rag" on me if any alarm sounded.

Some of the nurses tried to sound tough and some of the staff threatened to tie my wrists down. I disliked this very much, to put it mildly. There were times when I wanted to tear off the mask and throw it across the room.

I asked to see the doctor in charge to remedy my situation. I informed him that the equipment and people who ran the department needed to be more people-friendly. The mask needed to be soft and probably not army surplus from the 1917 biplane era. His staff needed to learn the words "please" and "thank you." I got good results from that little chat.

ANOTHER BETHESDA MIRACLE

Things improved, but my nights were racked with wacky dreams. One night I asked to see the head building engineer. I was convinced that they had me in the boiler room and sewer gas was coming up the drain in the floor. White squirrels and rats were in the wastebasket. I finally blamed all this nonsense on the goofy medicine in my system.

I continued to adjust to my new surroundings and make the best of my situation. My desire to be healed made me a survivor.

Chapter Seven
The Spanish Factor

Either in my hospital room or in therapy, I would always say a few words of greeting in Spanish to try to get a reaction from anyone who knew a few words of Spanish. One afternoon a man came into my room. I assumed he was on the housekeeping staff as he was sweeping and mopping the floor. I asked him in Spanish how it was going. ¿Qué passa? To my amazement he answered back in Spanish.

Everyone has a story. This guy was no exception. He was from Somalia in Africa, and was now living in the Twin Cities. As a young teen, while working in his father's store, he would wait on Cuban soldiers who were sent to Somalia in the 1970s to spread Castro's communist revolution. The soldiers would teach him some Spanish. You just never know when you need a little conversational Spanish!

One day a packet arrived from Santa Domingo where my friend, Mark DeJong, teaches fifth grade there in a Christian school. He had his students write me really nice cards and notes, all written in Spanish. Gracias, amigos!

I started to look forward more and more to mail time. Every day, about 1:00 P.M., I got mail, mostly from my students and the staff in Milaca.

Chapter Eight

Occupational, Physical and Speech Therapy

At Bethesda I began three main areas of therapy: physical, occupational, and speech therapy. For extra brain exercise, I would try and remember the head nurse's name on each shift. It helped keep the yogurt coming, even at two in the morning.

I remember Alice, the morning head nurse. Each day she would push open my door and say, "Barney, I'm praying for you." That got my day off to a good start.

In my room, I had to learn how to get from the edge of my bed into a wheelchair on the slide board, try to stand up, pivot, and sit. I had to recognize my array of medicines and what time of day or night I was to have what. It was up to me to buzz the head nurse to bring the right medicine and always monitor my blood pressure. I was to ask for a urinal or bedpan when I needed them.

I began work on building up my arm muscles. My schedule would be on the white board in my room. It would start with occupational therapy. Most every morning the occupational therapist would see to it that I could dress myself, brush my teeth, wash up, and get my pants, shoes and socks on. At this stage of rehab, I could not stand up or even get out of bed. I never knew that getting dressed could be so much work.

Good thing I didn't have to deal with a bra; just a tee shirt was a big enough job. My vision in my left eye wouldn't let me get it right. Finally, the occupational therapist showed me how to lay the shirt out on my lap so I could tell front from back and inside from outside. The shirts with a chest pocket were toughest. My vision and my brain just weren't doing things right. It became obvious I wouldn't be tying my own shoes anytime soon. Frustration city! I went the way of Velcro.

Then came the day I heard about a new bed that would do most everything –right. The control panel was two feet by two feet, crammed with buttons, bells and whistles. The West African gals had me moved in no time. One problem—no one, not even the head nurse, knew how to operate it.

The new bed had a depression in a certain location, which I could feel with my good right

Occupational, Physical and Speech Therapy

hand. I asked about it and was told it was for the bedpan. Their problem was no one could find the right-sized pan and no one could find the button to open the area for the bed pan. My problem was that I couldn't get to that spot without chest pain. And my left side was no help. I couldn't even sit up without the aid of a button on the bed. The power of suggestion with the bedpan got my bowels in motion. It was not pretty. The bed was no longer new—bedpan or not.

At first there was no solid food, just soups, broth and gelatin with fruit cocktail. The purchasing department must have found a real deal on fruit cocktail; it came with every meal.

During this stage of rehabilitation, my mind would digress to my days at Camp Roger, a summer youth camp in Michigan. During a fun campfire at the end of each session, the counselors would perform a wacky skit called "The Vipers." One person would come through the woods yelling, "The Vipers are coming, the Vipers are coming." Within a few seconds, two others would come running and yelling right up to the edge of the campfire, each carrying a roll of toilet paper. Then one of them would say loud enough for all to hear in the dark woods, "We are the Vipers." I needed the viper nurses quite often.

I was only a day or two into the Bethesda stay when I developed more and more of a problem eliminating water. It would hurt really bad just to try to pass water. If I couldn't get to a bathroom I realized someone had to put in a catheter somewhere along this journey. I complained to any nurse who would listen how badly it hurt to pee. There was a "mellow yellow" bag taped to my leg above the ankle somewhere.

I asked the nurse if they couldn't please do something because I had to try to roll a bit or move my legs to get water to pass. She came in with a big scissors and announced that the catheter from the first hospital must be getting plugged. (I never did figure what the big scissors was for.) She also announced that too much cinnamon in the system sometimes plugs them. I told her that I hadn't been to Tobie's in Hinckley for weeks for a cinnamon roll. So she decided to put in a newer, plastic model. I asked her if the one that was supposedly plugged was a bamboo Asian model. She didn't answer; she just gave a twist, a turn, and a tug to get it out. Now the water did flow with the plastic model. What relief!

When I could get around better, get out of bed and to the bathroom on my own, a nurse pulled the plastic model and the plumbing seemed to work just fine.

One morning the occupational therapist wanted to get me onto the portable commode, a device made of PVC pipe on wheels. She got me standing, into my wheelchair, and then we were to transfer from the wheelchair to the portable commode. While trying to back into the commode I bumped into it, tried to reach for the flimsy handrail, and lost my balance. I fell over backwards. The portable pot went sliding backwards and I went to the floor,

Occupational, Physical and Speech Therapy

while the occupational therapist was holding onto my gown.

Word quickly went out and before one could blink three times, a flurry of nurses and hospital workers were trying to get me right side up and back into the wheelchair. Four women couldn't budge me. Then the rehab doctor showed up, spun me around like a dial on a board game, and let me reach for a grab bar near the wash-up sink. I pulled myself up and the nurse shoved the wheelchair in back of me. So much for that experiment. Good thing the pot was empty. I begged them to take that thing away and not bring it back.

Soon after my transfer to Bethesda, the topic of solid food was brought up and how to handle the waste. I knew that in order to avoid the nursing home idea I would have to be able to handle all the bathroom functions, from top to bottom. The "Depends" route was tried for a couple of days, but definitely not the route to go. I decided I had to get up and get moving on my own. It took a while for my body to cooperate.

When I could get up and get into my wheelchair and wheel to the bathroom, I started practicing sitting on the throne and twisting and reaching with all my might to do the wiping thing. It wasn't easy since my rib cage still ached and my right arm wasn't long enough. But, alas! One day it happened. I could do it. I called the head nurse on my buzzer and broke the big news. Both good news and bad news spreads fast on the floor. I wanted to go to the bathroom all the time. Every time I saw a shadow anywhere near my door, I would yell, "Nurse, nurse, I did it!"

I sure was mouthy at times, and I was becoming a worse motor-mouth as the days passed. My son, David, tried staying overnight in the room with me just once. Never again. Imogene even tried sleeping in the chair in the room. She got zero sleep and so did I. The staff was irritated with my overnight antics.

I remember the day my rehab schedule started in earnest. The nurse who ran the Hoyer lift was summoned to lift me from the bed to a wheelchair. It was scary at first. I didn't want to trust the straps, rings and chains as they harnessed my hips and torso and pushed the lift button. Swinging in mid-air on that thing was no thrill. I hung on for dear life.

Their first goal was to get me to stand up by myself. I had a cast on my right leg, up to about the knee. At first I didn't realize all the signatures on it and I asked Imogene about how they got there. She filled me in on all of the visitors I had missed. Imogene explained to me that one of the names was Ann Kern. I never knew she was there. Mrs. Kern was the Milaca elementary principal at the time of the accident. To this day, Imogene can't say enough kind things about her being there when it mattered most. She was and is so grateful for Ann Kern.

Every day I worked at getting better. In the beginning, nurses would lift the bed, get me on the edge, and help me up. I couldn't even feel the floor with my left leg. It was scary. I figured I'd have to

Occupational, Physical and Speech Therapy

work overtime on my legs if I were ever to get out of that bed. So while I was in bed, I started to do leg lifts, which pulled on my stomach muscles. Even while awake at night I would practice. I knew I'd better get serious about getting my hip and stomach muscles going. Practice, practice, practice—chest pain or not! My right arm and hand were in good shape. I used them to help me lean forward.

From my wheelchair I also had to learn to use the smooth slide board to get from the chair to the elevated mats. They resembled wrestling mats. I would lie on my back while the therapist would attach small one- to two-pound weights on my ankles for more leg lifts with weights. I would work up a sweat every day. I would bring a sweat towel to physical therapy plus a plastic bottle with ice water. Why not go in style?

When at last I could stand up and slide on the smooth board between bed and wheelchair, I was promoted to the next grandiose contraption called the "light gait walker." While standing, the therapist would run straps through my legs and around my waist and chest, and lift me off the floor by pushing a button.

After the first day, I called it the "bungee machine." It took four therapists to run it: one ahead, one behind, and one on each side. Wouldn't you know I had visitors the first day they put me in this thing? They were Ralph and Marion Geddes from Burnsville. They went with me to therapy. I asked Ralph to carry my sweat towel and Marion carried my water bottle. What a sight! Only one leg would move and every few inches the therapist had to pull my left leg forward. I couldn't get it to do anything.

Every day the time I spent and distance I traveled on this thing would be extended, but, of course, there were not visitors every day. Imogene was, however, at my side for all therapy when she was in the building.

My left hand was a sight! When Imogene came to see me daily she would massage the left hand and fingers. Their natural color started to come back slowly and my fingers, minus the pointer, gained strength.

When the leg doctor gave permission to put some weight on the right leg, the therapists tried to get me to stand, even for a few seconds. I didn't think I could do it. My hip muscles on the left side wouldn't cooperate. I was numb all over. When I was able to put more weight on my right leg, life got a little easier. I would stand beside the bed, pivot and sit in the wheelchair.

My first major challenge was to get up and stand up from the wheelchair when I got to the therapy area. I didn't think I could ever do it. I thought I'd never walk again, even with a walker or a cane. I saw the ramps, steps, parallel bars, and other patients going through the routines. I soon realized I wasn't the only one there. It seemed there were new patients almost daily. Some were there because of accidents; others because of falls they had taken in their homes. My biggest heartache was listening to the cries and screams from young

Occupational, Physical and Speech Therapy

patients (teens) who were victims of four-wheeler accidents because they chose not to wear helmets.

I vividly remember my first steps. I got out of my wheelchair, stood up, balanced for a few seconds, and then I planned my next move if my legs would cooperate. The physical therapist sized me up with a walker. I was scared. My palms were wet with sweat. They actually wanted me to take the thing with two hands and take a few steps. I was petrified. At least with the podium walker on wheels I had something fairly stable to push and hang onto. The walker was much too light and flimsy.

I didn't realize it but everybody in the place was looking at me. My incessant jaw was quipping how I wouldn't be able to do this. Okay, here goes. Put your nose over your toes—uno, dos, tres—up we go. I got a hold of that walker, got the feel of it, tested the tennis ball no-skid feature on the tile floor, and started out. When I had gone just a few steps, the place erupted in cheering, applause and shouts. One comment I especially remember was, "Another Bethesda Miracle!"

Now that I had done this once, I worked at it again and again in future sessions. I learned had to sit up slowly or I would get dizzy. I would lean forward, do the nose-over-toes thing, then count to three. On the count of three I would struggle with all my might to push myself up with my good arm, with the wheelchair breaks on, and try to balance on my feet. A therapist would help on each side. It was a genuine accomplishment, but I knew more work lay ahead.

ANOTHER BETHESDA MIRACLE

As days progressed, I began to sense the miracle myself and often went to pieces because of it. The depression that comes with the type of stroke I had...well, let me just say, I wasn't ready for it. It hit me hard—would I ever walk again? Would I ever get back to my dear 650 Spanish students and the staff in Milaca?

A letter and card or a big envelope of mail would come and I'd go to pieces again. Just looking at the big banner they sent would get me off again. Families in the Milaca community would send letters, cards, and pictures of their family. This helped me focus on recovery.

The first thing every morning the occupational therapist would arrive and make sure I was dressed and ready for each trip to the big physical therapy session. I now had to slide myself on to a mat bench and do leg lifts to get warmed up a little. My other routine was to stay in the wheelchair and peddle the ergometer with my hands a certain number of times. The tension could be increased on it. All of these machines had counters, timers and buzzers so there was no lying about how long or how far or how many times around one went.

Oh, yes. There was also the stairs-stepper. My legs sure got a workout on that thing and the therapists could increase or decrease the tension to challenge one's muscles. Every day there was more and more time on the physical therapy machines.

Then came the day that they sized me up with the podium walker. At least I could lean on this podium-thing with wheels. I would hang on to two

Occupational, Physical and Speech Therapy

wooden handles that came out the top of it and try to walk in a straight line with my eyes on a certain goal across the room. It wasn't easy, but it got easier each time I tried it. I can honestly say that I never refused to at least try what they asked me to do.

Getting my left leg to slide ahead was a challenge. I had to learn to pick it up or my toe would catch and I would go down in a heap. Thankfully, I never took a serious tumble.

A mold of plastic was made for my left leg, which also had Velcro straps around my leg. What a pain! My shoe was supposed to go over that and be held in place with a special Velcro holder to keep the strings tight. To push my depression a notch further downhill, I was supposed to wear "teds," a tight stocking designed to help the swelling in my left leg. That didn't work well either. Everything was a struggle.

I got a nice surprise one Wednesday night in December. I had just taken a shower. I was in my wheelchair rolling down the hall to go back to my room with my gown flapping in the wind. That's when I saw George and Liz, a very dear couple from Arden Hills, Minnesota.

I was in the Peace Corps with them about

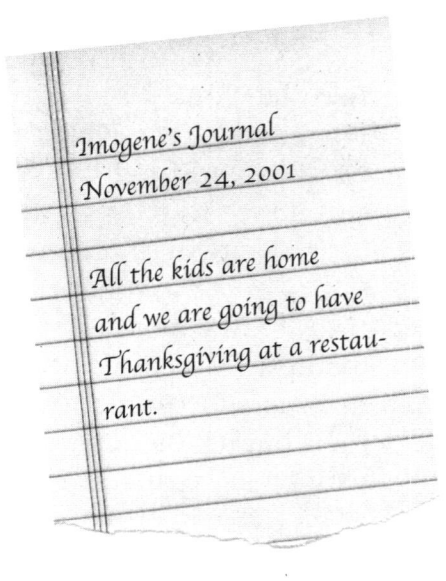

Imogene's Journal
November 24, 2001

All the kids are home and we are going to have Thanksgiving at a restaurant.

ANOTHER BETHESDA MIRACLE

forty years ago in Brazil. We had a lot of catching up to do, although we had seen each other and chatted on the phone from time to time over the years. Liz proceeded to chew me out royally for not letting them know sooner that I was in the hospital in St. Paul, just a few minutes from their home. Now when Liz chews, you know you got chewed.

This high school math teacher knows how to convey the power of ten. Liz used the Internet to contact as many of our old group as possible to tell them about me. Thirty-two of us had gone to Brazil together with a rural improvement program, something like 4-H Clubs. We traveled together at Arizona State University late in the summer of 1965. There we were trained in Portuguese by Brazillian instructors. We had to pass a physical endurance test which included walking down the Grand Canyon then out again the next day, which is a 14-mile hike one way.

> *Visitor's note*
>
> Bernie's dry humor was in full force during one of our visits to the hospital. Afterwards a nurse pulled us aside and asked, "Is Bernie always like this?"
> We assured her that he was just joking around.
>
> George & Liz Morse

After the nice, hot shower and a day of physical therapy, I was quite tired. Liz proceeded to tell me how, as a soccer mom, she would expect her son to blurt out ten blessings when the grumbling got too bad. I don't remember complaining about anything

Occupational, Physical and Speech Therapy

specific, but she decided not to leave the room until I verbally listed ten blessings. After all, it was the season to be thankful.

Liz said she would often wait at an intersection with the stoplights changing until she tallied ten blessings. I started listing my blessings: Imogene, Imogene, Imogene, Imogene, Imogene, Imogene, Imogene, Imogene, Imogene, and by number nine she stopped me. I had to be more creative, Liz said. I slept well that night.

My first get-well card from a Peace Corp crewmember came from Missouri. Yes, Judy, my coworker for two years, penned me a card. Here's what it said: "Bernie, I'm not praying for you. I'm praying for your nurses."

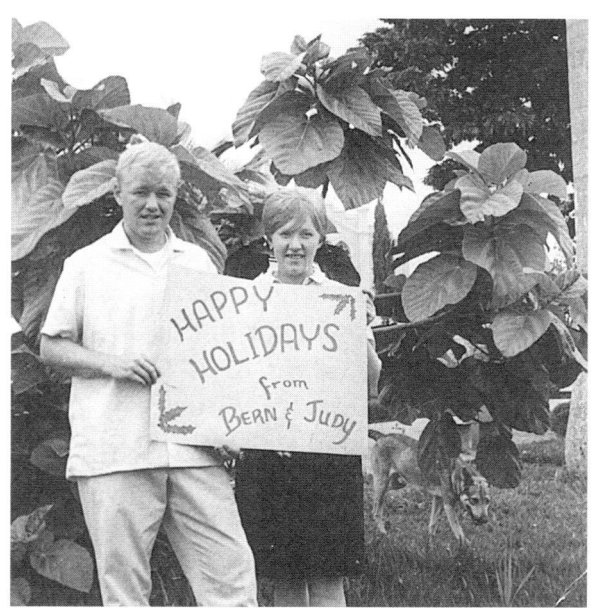

Bernie and Judy in Peace Corps, 1967

ANOTHER BETHESDA MIRACLE

All this time, I was also getting speech therapy. These sessions would involve the therapist asking some questions that were supposed to reveal how organized my brain was. My observation was that if I hadn't been organized for fifty-eight years, how would this bump make it any better?

Here are some sample questions. Name as many fruits as you can in one minute. On this one I tossed in several South American favorites like mango, papaya, and a couple of others that no one here in the United States has ever seen or tasted. Another question was to name as many vegetables as you can in one minute. I was also asked to name as many auto makers as I could. One particular session I was pitted against two other male patients in naming as many NFL quarterbacks past and present as I could. I'm not a big football fan, but I won that little contest rather handily.

One morning the therapist asked me what it means that you can lead a horse to water, but you can't make him drink. Now you readers must understand that I was a speech major at college in the 1960s. To answer that question, I asked the therapist if she had ever taken a calf to the county 4-H fair. Well, she was in for about a forty-minute dissertation about my taking my 4-H calf to the Kent County Fair in Michigan and how the critter would not drink the water and started to dehydrate. The chatter around the fair was that I was neglecting my calf and it was going to die because of dehydration. I had to call my dad to bring well water from the farm so my calf would drink. After this session I

Occupational, Physical and Speech Therapy

was informed that I would not have any more speech therapy.

As physical therapy continued, the occupational therapists were quite concerned with my left hand and arm. I couldn't lift my arm very far over my head. In occupational therapy one morning I had to balance a checkbook with about twenty entries. Then I had to study a batch of insurance quotes to find the best deal and coverage for the needs of a particular family.

During my stay, a couple of sixth graders really zapped me with their kindness and concern. Brock Welch wrote me a very kind note while I was in the hospital. Sarah Timmer showed off her determination and talent by making small items that were sold to raise funds for the taco dinner that I mentioned earlier.

> *Visitor's note*
>
> Hi. This is Brock Welch. I miss you and all the rest of sixth grade does too. I have been praying for you. I had a lot of people want me to say Hi to you. So Hi. I am sorry for what happened.
>
> Love, Brock Welch

During my years of teaching with elementary schools there was a sixth grader in Tillamook, Oregon, who came up with a question that for me takes first prize. Here's that story: We had welcomed a visitor one day who had just returned form a short mission trip to Indonesia. When the topic of food came up, and it always does with sixth graders, the guest explained that a real delicacy there was a boiled egg with a nearly full term chick inside. After the session, Billy C. raised a question. Did it taste more like a chicken, or more like an egg? We never got the answer. OK class, back to math.

When teaching in the classroom and when I was driving the bus, I always insisted on what I call "quick obedience," because slow obedience is disobedience. Trouble is, I flunked this test too many times in real life. Bethesda was no different. I got tested a lot. And often things did not go as planned.

In occupational therapy I was asked to move blocks and clothespins with my left hand. I was given a squeeze-pressure test with my left hand. Sometimes I had to build stacks of blocks and lift weights with my left hand. One morning my test in occupational therapy was to find the toaster, bread, and butter in the little kitchen and make myself some toast. Things were going well until I tried to spread the butter on the toast. Suddenly the toast went flying across the room, a victim of my left hand. I couldn't find the butter until I looked at my wheelchair. Wouldn't you know there was a glob of butter precisely on the adjustment bar for raising the footstep. It had always squeaked when it was adjusted, but not anymore. I used a napkin and greased up a few other areas, also—an old farmer has to use up the grease.

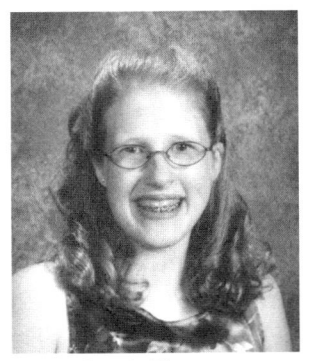

Sarah Timmer

Occupational, Physical and Speech Therapy

One late afternoon in late December two young Candy Stripers with a notepad and pencil in their hands appeared at my door and knocked gently. I invited them in. They had a question for me. "Are you Louie Anderson, the comic? You kind of look like him, and you sound like him." I said, "Girls, check the name by the door out there in the hall. As far as I know, I'm still old B. O., Bernie Oldenkamp from Hinckley, Minnesota." They left quickly with a smile.

Some families would come to visit me. I'll never forget them and their kindness. An early warning system informed me that a group of teachers was headed my way for a visit. I could hardly wait.

When friends and family came to visit during any of the physical therapy or occupational therapy time periods, I would always invite them to go with me. It was an afternoon session when my dear friend, Dick Case, came by for a visit. It turned out to be a memorable experience for both Dick and me!

I had to show Dick my stuff on the walker, going a few steps farther each time. Dick followed close behind, giving encouragement. My gray sweats started to sag more and more with each step and down they went, within

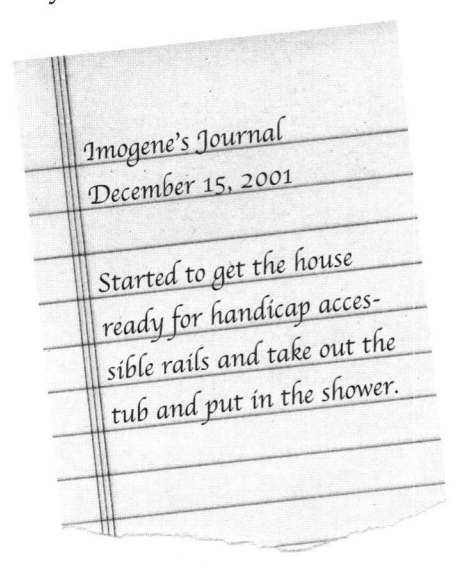

Imogene's Journal
December 15, 2001

Started to get the house ready for handicap accessible rails and take out the tub and put in the shower.

59

a full spectrum of therapist's patients and visitors. Before I knew it my sweats were around my knees. I didn't dare let go of the walker. I knew it and Dick let out a big holler. Here the guy was kind enough to come see me and I gave him a mooning we won't forget. Sorry again, Dick.

Later, Karen Baker from school came by the very hour I was to have a big "family" conference. On the agenda—my release from the hospital. I told the head nurse that she was from my school family, please let her in. And yes, she came along. Karen got the full scoop. My release date was set for January 6, 2002. Another milestone.

Three days before my release, the head physical therapist told me that I had to pass one major test. The test consisted of putting me down on the carpeted floor, next to a raised bed with a mat on it. I had to get on my hands and knees, get my torso up on the edge and somehow get into that bed. Our dear friends from St. James were there that day. I was nervous; I didn't think I could do it.

They put me on the floor. I got to my knees, amongst the cheers in the gallery. Then I got my

> *Imogene's Journal*
>
> *I see what a change this is going to be. How can I take care of him and still work? How will I be able to pay all the bills? I know that the Lord will help me. I have to trust Him, not myself.*

arms and elbows on the mat and started to spin with my right leg and lost my shoe. My left leg was quite worthless. I struggled and groaned. Then I got a surprise. My wife, Imogene, walked over, grabbed me by the seat of my sweats, tossed me on top of the raised mat and everybody cheered. I looked around and found I was now sharing a mat with a frail-looking little granny. I proudly announced to all spectators, "Look, Mom, I'm in bed with another woman!"

I passed.

Chapter Nine
A Christmas Visit

In anticipation of being released from Bethesda on January 6 of 2002, my doctor agreed to give me a personal leave day on Christmas of 2001. He wanted to see how I would do at home for a day and a night with my family. I was ready early because my wife is just never late (twenty-five years of driving school bus will do that to a person). The hospital staff got me in my wheelchair for the Christmas pass and got me to the waiting Caddy. The cold air felt so good. I did cover my nose for the transfer.

Imogene did really well on the Interstate I-35 system and on the St. Paul side streets, where the hospital is. I was surprised. But I also realized right away that maybe I should not be in the front seat. It

A Christmas Visit

was nerve racking. I should have gotten in the back with a grocery bag over my head. Life in the fast lane really made me nervous, especially at night. My mouth would get me in trouble riding with this million-mile mamma. Then my daughter Laura took over driving, and she demanded that I keep my mouth shut.

I survived Christmas day with the family. It went well. So after another "family meeting" my release date was confirmed and I was on my way. With bags packed I again headed for the main pickup area.

I kept the vow I had made earlier. When I arrived at the lobby I grabbed my walker, and yes, I did walk out of there. I would need more out-patient therapy in Sandstone, Minnesota, but I would not be in a nursing home. Maybe some day, but not yet.

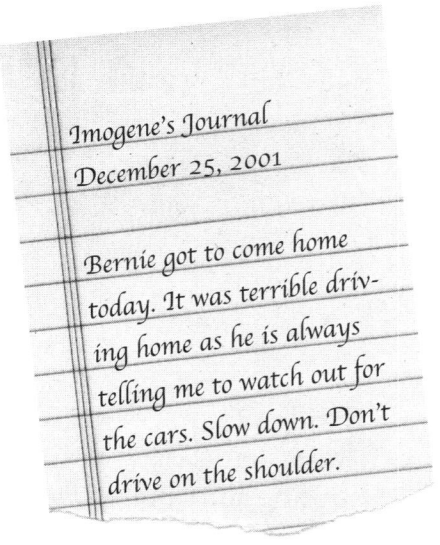

> *Imogene's Journal*
> *December 25, 2001*
>
> Bernie got to come home today. It was terrible driving home as he is always telling me to watch out for the cars. Slow down. Don't drive on the shoulder.

Imogene and Laura continued to make our little, on-a-slab house with no steps, more handicap-accessible.

Chapter Ten
A Miracle

I did not think of myself as a miracle the same way the Bethesda therapists did when they started hooting and hollering the day I took a couple of steps with the walker. Looking back, I guess it was a pretty big accomplishment getting this fifty-eight-year-old overweight guy out of bed without a lift, on his own feet, and moving on his own. The folks who saw me now as compared to the days and hours after the crash couldn't believe what or who they were looking at. More and more I heard the word "miracle" in the vocabulary of those around Bethesda.

A Miracle

Well, it wasn't luck; I can tell you that. The four-letter word "luck" was not to be used in our household growing up in the Old Dutch Reformed Church. What happened in our lives, for better or worse, was attributed to God's sovereignty being worked out—whether it was in the valley or on the mountain top, whether it was because of our own stupidity or someone else's, whether it was a life-giving or near-death situation.

It became a teaching opportunity when tragedy did strike, or a death or accident of some sort came our way. The Christian community would pull together, cite God's faithfulness, sing the great hymns of faith, review the Lazarus principal, use the bumps in the road to get more people saved and invite all who would listen to get themselves ready to meet their Maker at the Big House.

Through this accident and stroke I cannot claim a dramatic, near-death experience. No great light or tunnel or voices. The doctor at North Memorial told my wife that another five minutes along the way would have meant a different outcome. If the rescuers had

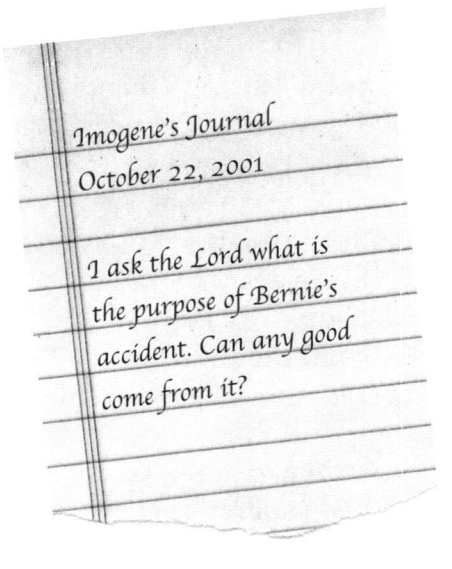

Imogene's Journal
October 22, 2001

I ask the Lord what is the purpose of Bernie's accident. Can any good come from it?

come five minutes later I wouldn't be here to tell you about this.

It's a common expression, "It wasn't my time yet." My Maker and Master Designer evidently has a bit of unfinished business with me. I'm not going to play dumb. If there is even one person who may read this and takes this blood pressure and stroke thing seriously, that may be reason enough.

I can still talk. In fact, I'm a worse motor mouth now than ever. There may undoubtedly come a day when the nursing home deal may be the way to go, but for now I have to move it or lose it.

The therapy was not easy, but I need to thank all of you who prayed and were such an encouragement. The words, "You can do it," or "Just hang in there" didn't always sit well with me, being the ornery Dutchman that I am. You were not in my shoes. But I became more determined to walk out of that hospital under my own steam. I realized that not all people do. I don't know why the guy across the hall from me didn't walk out. So what's the plan now? I'm not worried about it.

My heart goes out to others who have had the stroke experience. I realize that not all recover. I've been spared for a reason. I desperately desire to get back to my classroom in Milaca, but you don't need me on the road again with my vision the way it is.

Many real life miracles are recorded in Scripture. It may sound silly, but I'm thankful to be part of a big miracle. God takes a bunch of no-good, no-account bums, rescues them from hell through Jesus' blood and destines them to reign with Him

A Miracle

forever. With my sixty years on earth I'm starting to get it—the big picture. "We know that God causes everything to work together for the good of those who love God" (Romans 8:28a).

I must realize that God can do anything he chooses and I'll accept whatever he chooses. I can testify to the words of Psalm 77:14: "You are the God of miracles and wonders." I give God all the glory.

Chapter Eleven

The "61" Factor

I asked Imogene to call someone from my 1961 Rockford Senior High School graduating class. It didn't take long for the emails to start coming in, plus cards and phone calls. Our class had a bit of a complex. I'd call it the "nose in the air" class of the '60s at Rockford. It was commonly called "that class." We were known for our pranks and antics. Are we growing up? We're all 61 now. This class has been so loving and kind to me when they heard I was in the hospital. Just a bunch of good memories, they are! Thanks, class! I was the one who pulled the hinge-pins from Mr. Marvin's speech door. That

The "61" Factor

door sure was heavy—lucky Mr. Marvin didn't get crushed when it fell on him.

While I'm thanking special friends, thanks to you, Ken Van Loo, for your faithful phone calls. My Brazil Peace Corp group was so kind and positive. The students and staff at my former teaching locations in Alaska and Oregon also checked in. Also, a big thank you to Ruth Clark for the pillows for Laura and Imogene. Oh, you sweet ones. Our church family in Hinckley also did a benefit for us. We continue to make our little home more handicap-friendly inside and out.

While at Bethesda I came to realize that this stroke thing could really change things at whatever age, whatever size, and whatever background. Thanksgiving Day of 2001 brought my children, wife and grandson to my hospital room. My system was fairly well drugged up yet from my intensive care experience. My grandson, Joshua, was two years old. That triggered a story my mother would tell about me:

When I was two, my grandfather Bakker passed away while living at my parents' home. While I was toddling by his body lying on the couch, I tapped him on the arm and said in two-year old vocabulary, "Grandpa' sleeping." Grandpa had passed away of a massive stroke, it was believed. So now here I am. Still alive, reaching out to my grandson, who is two.

Before the accident, I was aware I was a good candidate for a stroke. My risk factors for stroke were adding up nicely: genetics, blood pressure, weight, sleep apnea, sedentary life style, not enough good exercise, and faulty diet. I had nearly every indicator that I was on my way to having a stroke. The problem was I did not get the message and make needed lifestyle changes. I was too busy, or so I thought, to take care of myself.

Chapter Twelve

Living With a Stroke

Before the stroke, I used to be able to go out and use the chain saw to cut wood and use the splitter for hours. I could move around and work all day. Now I have no balance to be able to handle a saw or a splitter. I am also afraid that I'll fall down.

I sometimes think I can do something as I sit in the house and think about it. But when I get outside right beside the task, like splitting wood with the hydraulic wood splitter, I find it too hard to handle. I tend to get more impatient and discouraged since the stroke.

ANOTHER BETHESDA MIRACLE

I find myself having a certain level of apathy with situations I used to care more about, like going to meetings. I often neglect people on my left side. A person may be standing at my left side, waiting to shake my hand, but I don't even notice them. I guess I'd better not drive on the highway with this disorder. One crash is enough.

In terms of dealing with depression, the drugs help, along with having supportive people around me. I'm finding out that, in my case, there is life after a stroke, thanks to the good help I get. I constantly try to think through projects I've started. That includes writing this account of my stroke and my recovery to this present moment.

One afternoon, when I was still at Bethesda, a letter arrived from a Milaca teacher. Now anyone reading this maybe has heard stroke survivors can get quite emotional over some things. The letter was so kind, gentle and caring that I went to pieces in a big way. The head nurse called in a counselor psychologist to deal with me. It led to another pill and anti-depressant. Yes, I kept a few of these types of letters.

Some folks just know how to touch an old stroke fella. There aren't many of these types of people around, but I'm blessed.

> **Imogene's Journal**
>
> I wish I could have someone to talk to, just to share my heart about all of this.

Chapter Thirteen

Mud and Mail

Once I was home, I was prone to go to the mailbox by whatever means possible to get the mail. My home nurse, Imogene, often gave me the you-be-careful-and-wear-underwear speech when she left at 1:00 P.M. for her afternoon bus run. I do spend from 6-9 A.M. and 1-5 P.M. home alone and fare quite nicely without any incidents. I try to be especially careful outside not to fall, always using my cane.

So on a muddy March 2003 afternoon I decided that I needed to get the mail, just down the driveway about 150 yards. I would take the truck (it's a four-by-four stick shift), but I could manage. I hung to the right just a bit too far and found myself stuck in the frost boil (soft spot) heading downhill toward the mailbox. My rear wheels were spinning, sinking more with each pop of the clutch. I would need to get out and lock the front hubs in four-wheel drive.

I got out with my cane and tried to hang on to the front of the truck. I first locked the left hub and made my way around in front, trying to hang on a bit to the bug shield to lock the hub on the passenger side. Mission accomplished, or so I thought. I started inching back to the driver's door. I tried to hang on to the front grillwork, but that ran out as I reached the driver's side. I grabbed for the groove along the hood but that was no help; my fingers wouldn't fit. The ground was soft and uneven. I felt my left shoe becoming stuck in the mud. I reached forward to try to reach the mirror bracket, but I was over-balanced and went to my knees.

I kept reaching for the mirror bracket hoping I could reach it to pull myself up, but every attempt only put me down further in the mud. I tried to get my right leg under me to reach and stretch. I had to use both hands and arms. On the third try I got partly up, but my sweats were very wet and soggy and heavy. All they would do is fall down. Oh, yes, Imogene did tell me to wear underwear, but, sorry, my mind started envisioning what time it was. Imogene wouldn't be home for two hours yet; everyone else was gone, thankfully. Imogene's sister was now living just fifty feet away. Again no

Mud and Mail

one home. Yelling wouldn't help. Why come and see the miracle old boy in the mud?

I resorted to stepping out of my sweats, not gracefully, and throwing them over the edge of the pickup box. I rescued one shoe and threw it in the box also. I could finally stand up, move ahead and get the driver's door open so I could get in. My feet were muddy, but at least I was up. A travel towel was on the seat, which I tried to spread out to keep at least some of the mud from my back and underside making the seat worse then wet.

Good thing the four-wheel drive worked. I continued on my journey, got the mail, made it back up the driveway and parked on the yard. What a mess! On my first trip in the house I rolled up the ugly wet sweats and dumped them and sweatshirt in the washer. I knew I'd have to pick rocks later. I got in the shower and watched the yellow-orange mud go down the drain. I figured I'd have to pick pebbles in the shower also, and spray that special cleaner on the walls and floor of the shower. I was very happy to be in the confines of our little house.

The pride was muddied up a bit as I waited for the lecture.

I called Imogene at the bus garage in town to ask a favor—to look for one of my shoes in the driveway on her way in.

Chapter Fourteen

A Tractor Ride

So what would an old farmer rather do? Just sit in the house on a fine spring sunny day or get out on his favorite toy and take a ride to the back forty and look things over after the long Minnesota winter?

Imogene put down a block of wood I could use as a step so I could get on my Kubota tractor. The year before, our land-clearing friend, Craig, made a couple of swipes through the woods where we flagged a trail for him to follow. We pushed a few stumps and rocks out of the way so the trail would be easier to follow in the future.

A Tractor Ride

I didn't think anything would slow down my four-wheel drive diesel tractor, but I've been wrong before. About fifty yards down the first new trail I found myself leaning to the left, and I was hanging on for dear life.

The tractor had slipped into a muddy hole where a large stump had been. All four wheels were spinning, but I went nowhere. I tried every maneuver that I knew of, but nothing worked. It wouldn't do any good to yell—I was too far from home. Imogene was already gone on her bus route. My son, Jeff, was working with the hydraulic log splitter. That little engine makes lots of noise. He would never hear me.

There was only one option, and that was to walk home, or at least as far as I could. I had carried my cane on the tractor. I slid off the tractor seat to the ground. Somehow I found enough solid ground and got on the trail to get out of there. It was very hard and I began to sweat. Little by little I got back to the main trail and walked a quarter mile back to our yard knowing I'd get a lecture for this outing. I had to call neighbor Monson to come with his big Oliver and hefty log chain to drag the Kubota backward with Jeff driving.

All right, more rules for the old man. No more tractor rides anywhere unless I told people where I was going, and how long I'd be gone and what my mission was going to be and what trail I would be on. OK, so I'm grounded. I got quite a bit of therapy that day, so I skipped my session the next morning as an outpatient in Sandstone.

Chapter Fifteen

Conrad Winslow

While I was in Bethesda, Imogene came one day with the mail from home. There was a cassette tape from a former student of mine from Homer, Alaska. She also brought a tape player.

The tape was from a former piano student. I didn't have Conrad in the first grade, but I remember Conrad as a thin-faced, shy six-year-old who begged his

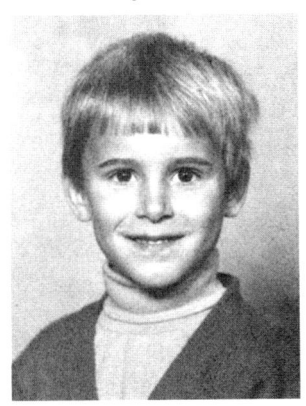

Conrad Winslow, age 6

Conrad Winslow

mother to let him try piano. On certain days after school I gave piano lessons for beginning students. Over the years, I've started out quite a few children on piano.

While sitting on the piano bench with me, Conrad's feet did not come close to touching the floor. After the first lesson I saw his smile. He had the smooth touch on the keyboard. When his mom came to pick him up I had but one observation. "He's got it," I said. "Keep him going somewhere."

Now Conrad has his own story to tell, and after listening to the tape he sent me while I was in rehabilitation, I hope you hear him make a piano talk sometime in a concert hall.

Conrad Winslow is now twenty years old and is a music major at Rollins College in Winter Park, Florida. He is also writing background music for new films soon to be released by independent filmmakers.

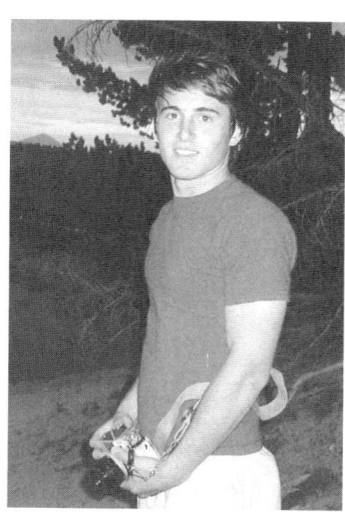

Conrad Winslow today

Chapter Sixteen

Saudades

This one word in Portuguese (pronounced Sow dah days) sums up my feelings towards all of you, wherever you are today, from Alaska to Argentina and east and west of these parts. Friends and family, far and near, when you ask me how I'm doing, don't be surprised if I give this answer: "Tengo" (I have) Saudades.

Saudades—a yearning, a craving, longing, hankering, yen, hunger, thirst, ache, very strong desire, fancy, wish I could see you all again, I wish I were with you, aspiration, anguish, passion, inclination, an intense homesickness. I miss you greatly.

Chapter Seventeen

A Visitor's View

This letter is written to share with you my memories of your accident, Bernie. It was an awful and sad day when our school learned of your accident. It was in October 2001, the beginning of the week. Thursday and Friday of that week school would be on vacation for state teacher's convention. Because of the anticipated recess, students were more active than usual. As was my custom, I was preparing for the 8:20 announcements. I received a phone call from the Superintendent's secretary telling me you had been in a serious car accident. I clearly understood you would not be in school that day, however, I did not know any more details. I immediately shared with the staff that you were in an accident and seriously injured.

As the morning proceeded, I received calls from your friends and wife, Imogene, telling us more details. I learned that you had a stroke while driving to work and hit a school bus head on. As I later learned, you were having difficulty getting ready for school that morning. You were unable to get your shirt on without assistance and were observed to be driving erratically. The accident with the bus resulted from your driving on the wrong side of the road. As we now know, you were experiencing a stroke.

I do know, Bernie, you are incredibly dedicated to your jobs of helping students. I say jobs because you were driving a school bus as well as teaching Spanish full time at Milaca Elementary. You were also the first to step forward and help with other teaching responsibilities as needed, such as after-school tutoring and subbing during your prep hour.

We learned, Bernie, that you were rushed to the local hospital and subsequently airlifted to North Memorial Medical Center in Robbinsdale. We were very fearful that you would not survive.

Later that week I came to the hospital to see you. I knew that you were unconscious and I would not be able to visit you. I wanted to bring you the many cards, banners and posters that the students had made for you. When you awoke, we wanted you to

A Visitor's View

see these messages and know of the hundreds who were thinking of you and sending prayers.

When I arrived at the hospital, I was nervous. I did not know what you would look like. You were in a circular ward. The ward had the nurses' station in the center with rooms in a circle around the station. Your door was open, and I could see your body lying on the bed. You were out. I believe Imogene was there. We spoke, and I left the written greetings form the staff and students.

You were unconscious for approximately one month. During that time I spoke with Imogene by phone to keep updated on your progress.

When you regained consciousness, Cheryl Warner and I visited on Saturday. We had a great visit. We were so thankful that you were alert and able to talk, like your old self. You were not able to be up and about, but certainly appeared to be recovering.

> *Visitor's note*
>
> *Hi. This is Doug. I miss you very much. I am sorry about what happened. 2nd grade misses you too. I am praying for you.*
>
> *love, Doug Welch*

I later learned that you did not remember our visit. That helped me better understand the seriousness of your injuries from the stroke.

The first Sunday after New Year's Day of 2002, my husband and I came through St. Paul and stopped to visit with you. I don't remember the name of the rehabilitation center, however, we

ANOTHER BETHESDA MIRACLE

did find it. We were so glad to see you! You were actually up and walked with the assistance of a walker. You were very optimistic that you would recover your physical strength and mental skills to be able to return to teaching a Milaca Elementary. I did not want to discourage you, but really wanted you to know that we did not want you to rush your recovery and have you return to work prematurely.

It was great day when you left rehabilitation and returned to Hinckley. I was not there to witness the event. I have had the good fortune to visit you several times since then.

I am sorry, Bernie, that you were not able to recover to the extent to allow you to return to teaching. You touched the hearts and lives of many students in Milaca. It has been a blessing for me to work with you too. Please know that you will always be in our hearts.

Sincerely yours,
Ann Kern
Former Principal,
Milaca Elementary School (1992-2003)

Chapter Eighteen

To My Students

Ever since my brain started to think a bit again after a month of intensive care in the hospital, I have had a hankering to sit down with all of you for a nice, long chat. I know you have questions to ask. That chat may not happen too soon, so I am anticipating what you may ask me.

Why can't I come back to teach some more? In short, my two main doctors won't let me. I can't drive anywhere. My left eye does not work very well and I can get very nervous just riding in a car or truck, especially at night.

ANOTHER BETHESDA MIRACLE

My speech is quite good. In fact, there are those who say I'm a worse motor mouth now than before. Can you imagine? I'm thankful that I did not lose my speech as some people do who experience a stroke.

My walking isn't the best, but at least I can get around with a cane. There was a time, as I lay in the hospital with a paralyzed left side and a broken right leg, I didn't think I would ever walk again.

So what is a stroke? I'll try to give you my take on this, but if you want to learn much more you can find lots of information on the Internet with the American Stroke Association.

A stroke is a disconnection. It's like part of your brain getting unplugged or injured by a blood clot which may have traveled to the brain from another part of the body. In my case, the doctors believe that part of my brain on my right side didn't get enough good, healthy blood with enough oxygen. Since the right side of your brain sends signals and messages to the left side of your head and body, the message box in your computer (brain) can't make good connections.

My left arm, left hand, left leg and foot do not have a normal feeling, even after three years. They feel a little numb, like what happens sometimes if you sit in one spot too long and your leg "goes to sleep," or so we say.

So when people ask me how I'm doing, I counter with another question. "Do your legs ever fall asleep?" The next question is, "Did they ever wake up?" My left side has not woken up totally yet. But

To My Students

after three years, I can now move my left ankle a little. To me, this is a big deal. As of Christmas 2004, I can even wiggle my left toes ever so slightly. I keep trying to move them every day and give them a workout!

So, do children ever have strokes? The answer is yes. There are many accounts of strokes in children. I try to read about them as much as possible. My first-ever contact with another stroke patient was back in 1985 when one of my teen Sunday School students was hospitalized in St. Paul with what was deemed to be a stroke. He was a very active thirteen-year-old, very normal, but collapsed on Easter Sunday afternoon in his backyard in Hinckley while playing touch football with family and friends. I went to see Barry in the hospital. Weeks later I heard him sing, "I Am a Possibility" in church. There was not a dry eye in the place. Barry now has a lovely family and resides in the Twin Cities area. He was, and is, a great inspiration.

Now this old Señor teacher is going to give all you students, older and younger, and families, some advice which you've heard before. First of all, when in doubt about the danger of an activity, wear a helmet. While I was in therapy in the hospital for older people (not children), I heard the screams and cries from the patients who thought they knew everything and went on the toys, snowmobiles, four-wheelers, and so on, with no head protection. A head injury can cause a stroke on the spot if the brain is injured with a bump. Second, please do not

ANOTHER BETHESDA MIRACLE

play dangerous games by trying to make each other faint. Do not be estupido.

Can people tell if they are going to have a stroke? That's a tough question. Every time you see the doctor they usually take your blood pressure, even if you're a youth. If there is high blood pressure, or a history of high blood pressure in your family, listen to your doctor and get help.

Stroke is often called the silent or stealth killer. Well, it sure can mess up your life. If your hand, leg, arm or foot tingles, get it checked out, sooner rather than later. Headaches without any good reason are another clue. If I had listened to one warning signal, it would have helped. We have just one life, take necessary care of it. It will be worth the effort.

But, we go forward with "Faith in God and your foot on the floorboard," as we said in Brazil. We did have a vehicle in Brazil we named "Jesus is calling." It was a Volkswagen van with basically no protection in front of the driver. If you were in an accident, it was over. Good thing I was driving a Buick.

As most of my former students may agree, Señor Oldenkamp was sure a "bear" about respect, responsibility, and fresh air. Okay, I admit I may have been the grouch of the universe at times, but I would not tolerate disrespect of any size, shape or form in the classroom, or anywhere in school or on the bus.

That lousy Spanish folder was only a small exercise in being responsible. Thanks for coming to class with a folder.

To My Students

While in the hospital, my mind went back a few years (about forty-five years) to a 4-H ceremony in Kent County, Michigan, where I received the county "I Dare You" award for that year. I received the "I Dare You Book" published by the Danforth Foundation. I read it cover to cover. I suggest you find a copy sometime and read it.

I learned from that book that when given a choice of where to walk down the street when it's 100 degrees in the shade, always walk on the sunny side of the street with a big smile and say "Good day" to everyone you meet, friend or foe.

Stand tall, suck in the gut, shoulders back, chest out, chin down, mean business, sit up straight, and please don't mumble to me.

"Let's have more fresh air." I contend that elementary classrooms need more fresh air for better learning. More oxygen for the brain! When I would come to visit some of your classrooms I would have to leave. There wasn't enough good air for all of us.

Chapter Nineteen

The Faith Factor

That first month in intensive care brought several of you to my bedside. I thank you. I understand that some of you walked away, shaking your head. Would any amount of faith or prayer pull this guy through? I wasn't with the program myself; all I remember from the accident was the lights in front of me and the big air bag. When my mouth started running again, maybe it never stopped. I'm told that I asked visitors if they had a plan to get me out of there. I didn't have a plan, but it looks like God did. On His watch it wasn't my time, although later I learned that a doctor there told Imogene I had made it by only five minutes.

Now after three years of being home, I can still get up in the morning asking, "What's your plan today, Lord?" It wasn't until that moving day from North Memorial Hospital to Bethesda that I came to my senses enough to know the Lord and I needed to do some serious talking. Even the slightest thought of not getting back to my students was crushing.

I slipped into a depression, but got help from professionals on the hospital staff. I begged for the hospital chaplain to come by, talk and pray. We did! I cried loud and long over every letter from Milaca and from family.

On one of my hometown pastor's visits, I asked him to read from John, chapter five, where Jesus walked by a bunch of paralytic cripples waiting by the pool for the water to be stirred. I now was one of them, and when Jesus asked, "Do you want to be healed?" my hand was up. I didn't care what day healing would come or how many months or years it would take, but I knew then, and I know now, that He is the Healer.

The total job will get done when that resurrection trumpet sounds. So it looks like I'll have to hang

> *Visitor's note*
>
> Bernie,
>   Can't leave us yet. Still need help with spelling and life in general. (Praying for you.)
>
> Love,
> John Rakin, Tracy & Family

ANOTHER BETHESDA MIRACLE

around, reviewing the Westminster and Heidelberg Catechism, and all of Scripture, pointing all the hurting and crippled folks to the One who does the big miracle the hour you and I open our hearts to Him. So lets stop bickering. Let's get this barbaric generation saved and shipped on to glory when He calls.

I've done quite a few funeral sermons in my years with the Mission. The funerals are not always easy, but with the families who have seen the Big Picture and walk by faith along life's trail, it's always so comforting to get to the hope we have in Jesus.

When there is a tragedy or sickness, we Christians grab the Scripture and take the refresher course in the Lazarus Principle from John 11:4. This sickness is not unto death, but for the glory of God.

I will not begin to surmise who had the greater faith with getting me up and running again after the "bump." Was it my faith, or the faith of those who came and laid hands on me? Or maybe it was the faith of all those who stayed at home in their own prayer chambers and in their own way prayed for me. Was it the heavy hitting prayer of the pastors, or the simple expressions of those 1st graders? God's decision is final. I thank Him first, and thank all of you who thought of me along the way. Keep it up. More miracles are coming.

About the Author

Bernie Oldenkamp is a native of Rockford, Michigan, and a graduate of Calvin College. He spent three years as a Peace Corp volunteer in Brazil in the late 1960s. He returned to the states for a year to teach at a Christian school in New Holland, South Dakota.

For most of the 1970s, Bernie spent time as a lay missionary in Brazil. He returned to the states once again and taught at another Christian school in Sandstone, Minnesota. He obtained his bachelor of science degree and his Minnesota teaching certificate for kindergarten through sixth grade from Northwestern College in St. Paul in 1991. He continued teaching in such places as Homer, Alaska; Tillamook, Oregon; and Onamia and Milaca, Minnesota. He was also a licensed auctioneer, where he could talk as fast as he wanted.

Mr. Oldenkamp has been unable to teach since the stroke and the accident, but continues to use his Spanish skills when friends come calling. He and his wife Imogene have four grown children and make their home in Hinckley, Minnesota.